Breast Cancer Diet Cookbook For Newly Diagnosed

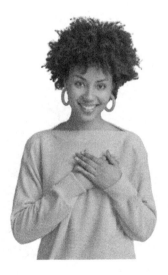

A Cookbook for Newly Diagnosed Warriors to Repair, Regenerate & Detoxify

Dr. Lucy Mogen

Copyright © Lucy Mogen 2023

ALL RIGHTS RESERVED. No part of this report may be modified or altered in any form whatsoever, electronic, or mechanical, including photocopying, recording, or by any informational storage or retrieval system without express written, dated and signed permission from the author.

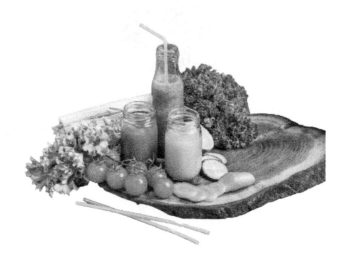

Contents

Contents 3

INTRODUCTION 9

Chapter 1 14

    The Basics of a Breast Cancer Diet 14

    Foods to Avoid in a Healthy Breast Cancer Diet 17

Chapter 2 24

    Morning Magic: Wholesome and Energizing Recipes to Start Your Day 24

        1. Blueberry Oat Muffins 24

        2. Morning Frittata 25

        3. Avocado Toast 27

        4. Overnight Oats 28

        5. Egg and Veggie Breakfast Burritos 28

        6. Quinoa Fruit Bowl 30

        7. Sweet Potato Toast 31

        8. Smoothie Bowl 32

        9. Breakfast Tacos 33

        10. Baked Oatmeal 34

Chapter 3 36

    Lunchtime Bliss: Delicious and Nutritious Recipes to Fuel Your Day 36

        1. Sweet Potato and Black Bean Burrito Bowl 36

- 2. Mediterranean Quinoa Salad 37
- 3. Roasted Vegetable and Chickpea Bowl 38
- 4. Spinach and Artichoke Stuffed Portobello Mushrooms 39
- 5. Curried Cauliflower Rice Bowl 40
- 6. Cucumber and Avocado Salad 41
- 7. Baked Tofu and Vegetable Skewers 42
- 8. Mediterranean Chickpea Salad 43
- 9. Mediterranean Farro Bowls 44
- 10. Asian Noodle Bowls 45

Chapter 4 47

Nourishing Plates: Delicious Dinners for Breast Health 47

- 1. Mediterranean Salmon with Spinach: 47
- 2. Roasted Asparagus with Mushrooms: 48
- 3. Baked Sweet Potato Fries: 49
- 4. Grilled Chicken with Avocado Salsa: 50
- 5. Grilled Zucchini and Squash: 51
- 6. Roasted Brussels Sprouts and Butternut Squash: 51
- 7. Quinoa and Kale Salad: 52
- 8. Grilled Portobello Mushrooms: 53
- 9. Roasted Broccoli and Cauliflower: 54
- 10. Grilled Vegetable Skewers: 54

Chapter 5 57

Bites of Strength: Snacks & Appetizers to Empower Breast Cancer Warriors 57
1. Roasted Asparagus with Parmesan 57
2. Avocado Toast 57
3. Baked Sweet Potato Fries 58
4. Veggie Quesadillas 59
5. Hummus and Veggie Platter 60
6. Baked Zucchini Fritters 60
7. Mediterranean Tuna Salad 61
8. Mediterranean Yogurt Dip 62
9. Broiled Salmon with Garlic and Herbs 63
10. Roasted Brussels Sprouts 64

Chapter 6 65

Desserts & Treats for Hope: Scrumptious Sweets to Uplift and Inspire Newly Diagnosed Breast Cancer Warriors 65

1. Apple and Cinnamon Oatmeal Crumble Bars 65
2. Coconut Chia Seed Pudding 66
3. Sweet Potato Brownies 67
4. Banana Oat Cookies 68
5. Raspberry Coconut Chia Popsicles 69
6. Chocolate Coconut Macaroons 70
7. Baked Apples with Walnuts and Raisins 71
8. Pear Crisp 72
9. Blueberry Coconut Oat Bars 73

10. No-Bake Coconut Date Balls 74

Chapter 7 77

Pink Blends: Delicious Juice & Smoothie Recipes for a Healthy Journey 77

1. Strawberry Banana Smoothie 77
2. Green Protein Smoothie 77
3. Pineapple Coconut Smoothie................................ 78
4. Carrot Apple Smoothie.. 79
5. Green Detox Smoothie 79
6. Beet Citrus Smoothie.. 80
8. Berry Spinach Juice.. 81
10. Creamy Coconut Smoothie 82

Chapter 8 83

Heartful Bowls: Veggie Recipes for Newly Diagnosed Breast Cancer Thrivers 83

1. Roasted Butternut Squash, Brussels sprouts, and Chickpeas: 83
2. Zucchini Noodle Salad with Avocado: 84
3. Roasted Sweet Potato and Red Pepper Soup: 85
4. Quinoa and Kale Power Bowl: 86
5. Roasted Broccoli, Carrots, and Chickpeas:.......... 87
6. Spicy Black Bean and Quinoa Bowl: 88
7. Baked Eggplant and Chickpea Curry: 89
8. Roasted Cauliflower and Chickpea Bowl:............. 90
9. Kale and Avocado Salad:...................................... 91

- 10. Quinoa and Roasted Veggies Bowl: 92

Chapter 9 95

Green for Hope: Delicious Salads Recipes for Newly Diagnosed Breast Cancer Fighters 95

- 1. Broccoli and Tomato Salad: 95
- 2. Avocado and Spinach Salad: 96
- 3. Kale and Roasted Sweet Potato Salad: 96
- 4. Quinoa and Black Bean Salad: 97
- 5. Roasted Beet and Feta Salad: 98
- 6. Carrot and Chickpea Salad: 99
- 7. Cucumber and Tomato Salad: 99
- 8. Apple and Walnut Salad: 100
- 9. Zucchini and Feta Salad: 101
- 10. Quinoa and Apple Salad: 102

Chapter 10 103

Stronger Together: Nutritious and Flavorful Sides Recipes for Fighting Breast Cancer 103

- 1. Lentil and Squash Stew with Cumin-Roasted Chickpeas 103
- 2. Broccoli and Quinoa Salad 105
- 3. Kale and Roasted Beet Salad 106
- 4. Zucchini Noodle Bowl with Garlic-Miso Sauce ... 107
- 5. Quinoa Cakes with Spinach and Feta 108
- 6. Sweet Potato and Chickpea Curry 109
- 7. Grilled Eggplant and Zucchini with Rosemary 110

8. Roasted Cauliflower and Chickpea Bowl............ 111

9. Roasted Vegetable and Couscous Bowl 112

10. Roasted Carrot and Lentil Salad 114

Chapter 11 117

Bowlfuls of Bravery: Delicious & Heartwarming Soups for Breast Health 117

1. Roasted Tomato and Red Pepper Soup 117

2. Creamy Carrot Soup 118

3. Cauliflower and Leek Soup 119

4. Lentil Soup 120

5. Asparagus Soup 121

6. Kale and White Bean Soup 123

7. Broccoli and Cheddar Soup 124

8. Butternut Squash Soup 125

9. Parsnip and Potato Soup 126

10. Sweet Potato and Cumin Soup 127

Chapter 12 129

30 Days Culinary Crusade for Newly Diagnosed Breast Cancer Fighters 129

Conclusion 141

INTRODUCTION

Edna had always been a vibrant and energetic woman. She loved life and all its challenges, and she faced them head-on. But when she was diagnosed with breast cancer, her world came crashing down.

At first, Edna was devastated. She couldn't believe that this was happening to her. But then she decided that she wasn't going to let cancer defeat her. With everything she had, she was going to fight it.

Edna knew that she needed to make some serious changes to her lifestyle. She had always been a bit of a foodie, indulging in rich and delicious meals whenever she could. But now she realized that her diet needed to change. She started eating more fruits and vegetables, and she cut out all the processed foods and sugary drinks.

At first, it was tough. Edna missed her old favorite foods. But she soon realized that she was feeling better than she had in years. Her energy levels were up, and her body felt strong. She knew that her new diet was helping her fight cancer.

Edna also made some other lifestyle changes. She started exercising more regularly, taking long walks in the park and practicing yoga. She found that these activities helped her feel calm and centered, even when things were tough.

Of course, Edna's treatment wasn't just about diet and lifestyle changes. She also underwent chemotherapy, which was tough on her body. But she stayed positive and focused, knowing that the chemo was an important part of her recovery.

Throughout it all, Edna stayed connected with her loved ones. She leaned on her family and friends for support, and they were always there for her. She also joined a support group for breast cancer survivors, where she found comfort and inspiration from others who had gone through the same thing.

Months went by, and Edna's strength and determination paid off. Her cancer was in remission. She was overjoyed, but she also knew that she couldn't let her guard down. She continued to eat healthily, exercise, and stay connected with her support network.

Years passed, and Edna stayed cancer-free. She knew that she had overcome breast cancer through a combination of different strategies: diet, lifestyle changes, chemo, and emotional support. She felt grateful for every day and lived life to the fullest.

Today, Edna is a beacon of hope for others who are going through the same thing. She shares her story with others, inspiring them to take charge of their health and never give up. She knows that the journey isn't easy, but she also knows that it's worth it. Because in the end, there's nothing more precious than life itself.

Breast cancer can simply be described as the type of cancer that affects the cells of the breast. It is the most commonly diagnosed cancer among women in the United States.

According to the Centers for Disease Control and Prevention, breast cancer is the second leading cause of death for women in the United States. About one in eight women in the United States will be diagnosed with breast cancer in their lifetime.

In the United States alone, there were an estimated 276,480 new cases of invasive breast cancer in women in 2019. Additionally, there were 48,530 new cases of non-invasive breast cancer in women. Unfortunately, an estimated 42,170 women in the United States died from breast cancer in 2019.

The second most prevalent disease overall and the most common cancer in women worldwide is breast cancer. It is estimated that over 2.1 million women were diagnosed with breast cancer in 2018. Additionally, 627,000 women died from breast cancer in 2018.

Nutrition plays an important role in the prevention and treatment of breast cancer. Eating a healthy diet can help reduce the risk of developing breast cancer, as well as improve outcomes for those who have been diagnosed with the disease. Eating a balanced diet full of fruits, vegetables, whole grains, and lean proteins can help reduce the risk of breast cancer and improve outcomes for those who have been diagnosed with the disease.

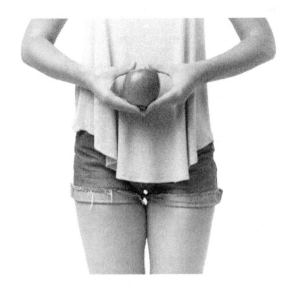

Chapter 1

The Basics of a Breast Cancer Diet

Breast cancer has been known to be a serious and potentially life-threatening disease that affects millions of women worldwide. While there is no one-size-fits-all approach to treating breast cancer, research has shown that a healthy diet can help reduce the risk of developing the disease, support the immune system during treatment, and aid in recovery and survivorship.

In this article, we will provide an overview of a healthy breast cancer diet, including the foods to include and avoid, nutrient requirements, and the importance of hydration.

Foods to Include in a Healthy Breast Cancer Diet

A healthy breast cancer diet should include a variety of nutrient-dense foods that provide essential vitamins, minerals, and antioxidants to support the immune system and overall health. Here are some of the foods to include in a healthy breast cancer diet:

Fruits and Vegetables

Fruits and vegetables are rich in antioxidants and phytonutrients that can help reduce the risk of developing breast cancer and support the body's immune system during treatment. Aim to consume at least five servings of fruits and vegetables per day, including a variety of colors, such as green leafy vegetables, orange and yellow vegetables, and red and purple fruits.

Whole Grains

Whole grains are a good source of fiber, which can help maintain a healthy weight and reduce the risk of breast cancer. Whole grains include foods such as brown rice, quinoa, oatmeal, and whole wheat bread.

Lean Protein

Lean protein sources, such as fish, chicken, turkey, and legumes, can help maintain muscle mass and support the immune system during treatment. Plant-based proteins, such as tofu and tempeh, are also good choices for a healthy breast cancer diet.

Healthy Fats

Healthy fats, such as those found in nuts, seeds, avocados, and fatty fish, can help reduce inflammation and support heart health. However, it is essential to consume healthy fats in moderation, as they are high in calories.

Low-fat Dairy

Low-fat dairy products, such as milk, yogurt, and cheese, are good sources of calcium and vitamin D, which are essential for bone health. However, it is crucial to choose low-fat or non-fat dairy products to reduce saturated fat intake.

Water

Staying hydrated is crucial for overall health and is especially important during breast cancer treatment. Aim to drink at least eight glasses of water per day, or more if you are physically active or live in a hot climate.

Foods to Avoid in a Healthy Breast Cancer Diet

A healthy breast cancer diet should also avoid foods that can increase the risk of cancer or interfere with treatment. Here are some of the foods to avoid in a healthy breast cancer diet:

Processed Foods

Processed foods, such as fast food, chips, and candy, are high in calories, saturated fat, and sodium, and can contribute to weight gain and increase the risk of cancer. Instead, and if possible, choose whole, minimally processed foods.

Red and Processed Meats

Red and processed meats, such as beef, pork, and bacon, have been linked to an increased risk of cancer. Instead, choose lean protein sources, such as fish, chicken, turkey, and legumes.

Sugary Drinks

Sugary drinks, such as soda and fruit juice, are high in calories and can contribute to weight gain and increase the risk of cancer. Instead, choose water, herbal tea, or unsweetened beverages.

Alcohol

Alcohol consumption has often been associated with an increased risk of breast cancer. It is best to limit alcohol consumption or avoid it altogether during breast cancer treatment.

Nutrient Requirements for a Healthy Breast Cancer Diet

A healthy breast cancer diet should provide adequate nutrients to support the immune system and overall health. Nutrient requirements for a healthy breast cancer diet include a balance of macronutrients (carbohydrates, protein, and fat) and micronutrients (vitamins and minerals). Adequate hydration is also essential for overall health and during cancer treatment. Here are some key nutrients to focus on when planning a healthy breast cancer diet:

Protein

Protein is essential for building and repairing tissues, including muscles and organs. During cancer treatment, protein is also needed to support the immune system and aid in recovery. Aim to consume at least 0.8 grams of protein per kilogram of body weight per day, or more if you are physically active or undergoing cancer treatment.

Good sources of protein include poultry, fish, lean meats, eggs, dairy products, legumes, nuts and seeds.

Carbohydrates

Carbohydrates are the body's main source of energy and are needed for physical activity and brain function. However, it is essential to choose complex carbohydrates, such as whole grains, fruits, and vegetables, over simple carbohydrates, such as sugar and refined grains.

Aim to consume at least 130 grams of carbohydrates per day, or more if you are physically active.

Fat

Fat is essential for the absorption of certain vitamins and minerals, and also plays a role in hormone production and cell growth. However, it is important to choose healthy fats, such as those found in nuts, seeds, avocados, and fatty fish, and limit saturated and trans fats.

Aim to consume no more than 20-35% of your daily calories from fat, with a focus on healthy sources.

Calcium and Vitamin D

Calcium and vitamin D are essential for bone health and can help reduce the risk of osteoporosis, a common side effect of breast cancer treatment. Good sources of calcium include low-fat dairy products, leafy green vegetables, and fortified foods, such as orange juice and cereal. Sunlight exposure, fortified foods, and supplements are all sources of vitamin D.

Aim to consume 1,000-1,200 milligrams of calcium per day and 600-800 international units of vitamin D per day.

Iron

Iron is essential for the production of red blood cells and can help prevent anemia, a common side effect of cancer treatment. Good sources of iron include lean meats, poultry, fish, legumes, and fortified cereals.

Aim to consume at least 18 milligrams of iron per day, or more if you are a premenopausal woman.

Hydration

Staying hydrated is crucial for overall health and is especially important during cancer treatment. Aim to drink at least eight glasses of water per day, or more if you are physically active or live in a hot climate.

A healthy breast cancer diet should include a variety of nutrient-dense foods that provide essential vitamins, minerals, and antioxidants to support the immune system and overall health. The diet should also limit foods that can increase the risk of cancer or interfere with treatment.

By focusing on nutrient-rich foods, maintaining a healthy weight, staying hydrated, and avoiding alcohol, individuals can support their overall health and well-being during and after breast cancer treatment. Consulting with a registered dietitian can also provide individualized guidance and support for a healthy breast cancer diet.

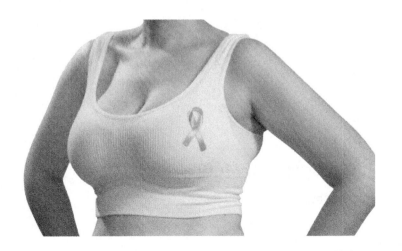

Chapter 2

Morning Magic: Wholesome and Energizing Recipes to Start Your Day

1. Blueberry Oat Muffins

Ingredients:
- 2 cups flour
- 2 cups rolled oats
- ½ cup coconut sugar
- 2 teaspoons baking powder
- ½ teaspoon baking soda
- ½ teaspoon salt
- 2 teaspoons ground cinnamon
- 2 eggs
- ½ cup vegetable oil
- 1 cup almond milk
- 2 teaspoons vanilla extract
- 2 cups fresh blueberries

Instructions:

1. Preheat oven to 350°F (175°C) and lightly grease a muffin pan with non-stick cooking spray.
2. In a large bowl, whisk together the flour, oats, sugar, baking powder, baking soda, salt, and cinnamon.
3. In a separate bowl, mix together the eggs, oil, almond milk, and vanilla extract.
4. Wet ingredients should be added to the dry ingredients, and stir until just combined.
5. Gently fold in the blueberries.
6. Divide the batter evenly among the 12 muffin cups.
7. Bake for 20-25 minutes, or until a toothpick inserted into the center of a muffin comes out clean.
8. Let cool for ten minutes before transferring to a cooling rack.

2. Morning Frittata

Ingredients:
- 4 eggs
- ½ cup skim milk
- ¼ teaspoon salt
- ¼ teaspoon ground black pepper
- ½ cup cherry tomatoes, diced

- ½ cup red bell pepper, diced
- ¼ cup red onion, diced
- ½ cup cooked, shredded chicken
- Approximately 2 tablespoons chopped fresh herbs (such as basil, parsley or thyme)
- 2 tablespoons olive oil

Instructions:
1. Preheat the oven to 375°F (190°C).
2. Whisk the eggs, milk, salt, and pepper in a medium bowl.
3. Heat the olive oil in a large oven-safe skillet or pot, and over medium heat.
4. Add the tomatoes, bell pepper, onion, chicken, and herbs and cook for 5 minutes, stirring occasionally.
5. Pour the egg mixture over the vegetables and cook for 5 minutes, stirring occasionally.
6. Place the skillet in the oven and bake for 15-20 minutes, or until the frittata is golden brown and a toothpick inserted into the center comes out clean.
7. Let cool for 10 minutes before serving.

3. Avocado Toast

Ingredients:
- 2 slices whole grain bread
- ½ cup mashed avocado
- 1 teaspoon olive oil
- ¼ teaspoon salt
- ¼ teaspoon ground black pepper
- 2 tablespoons crumbled feta cheese
- 2 tablespoons diced tomatoes
- 2 tablespoons diced red onion
- Two tablespoons of chopped fresh herbs such as parsley, basil, or thyme.

Instructions:

1. Toast the bread in a toaster or in a preheated oven at 350°F (175°C) for 5 minutes.
2. In a small bowl, mash together the avocado, olive oil, salt, and pepper.
3. Spread the mashed avocado on the toast slices.
4. Top with the feta cheese, tomatoes, red onion, and herbs.
5. Serve immediately.

4. Overnight Oats

Ingredients:

- ½ cup rolled oats
- ½ cup almond milk
- 1 tablespoon chia seeds
- 1 tablespoon honey
- ½ teaspoon ground cinnamon
- ¼ cup plain Greek yogurt
- ¼ cup fresh blueberries
- ¼ cup sliced almonds

Instructions:

1. In a bowl, mix together the oats, almond milk, chia seeds, honey, and cinnamon.
2. Cover and refrigerate overnight.
3. In the morning, stir in the Greek yogurt and top with the blueberries, almonds, and additional honey, if desired.
4. Serve chilled.

5. Egg and Veggie Breakfast Burritos

Ingredients:

- 4 whole wheat tortillas
- 4 eggs
- ½ cup skim milk
- ¼ teaspoon salt
- ¼ teaspoon ground black pepper
- ½ cup diced bell peppers
- ½ cup diced tomatoes
- ¼ cup diced red onion
- ¼ cup cooked, shredded chicken
- 2 teaspoons of fresh herbs, chopped (such as parsley, basil, or thyme)
- 2 tablespoons olive oil
- ¼ cup grated cheese

Instructions:
1. Heat a large pot over medium heat.
2. In a bowl, whisk together the milk, eggs, salt, and pepper.
3. Add the olive oil to the skillet.
4. Add the bell peppers, tomatoes, onion, chicken, and herbs and cook for 5 minutes, stirring occasionally.

5. Pour the egg mixture into the skillet and cook for 5 minutes, stirring occasionally.

6. Divide the egg mixture among the 4 tortillas and top with the grated cheese.

7. Roll up the tortillas and serve.

6. Quinoa Fruit Bowl

Ingredients:

- 2 cups cooked quinoa
- 2 tablespoons honey
- 1 teaspoon ground cinnamon
- ¼ cup plain Greek yogurt
- ¼ cup diced fresh fruit (such as strawberries, blueberries, or blackberries)
- 2 tablespoons chopped nuts (such as almonds, walnuts, or pecans)
- 2 tablespoons shredded coconut

Instructions:

1. In a large bowl, mix together the cooked quinoa, honey, and cinnamon.

2. Divide the quinoa mixture among 4 bowls.

3. Top each bowl with the Greek yogurt, fruit, nuts, and coconut.

4. Serve immediately.

7. Sweet Potato Toast

Ingredients:

- 2 sweet potatoes, sliced lengthwise into ½-inch (1 cm) slices
- 2 tablespoons olive oil
- ¼ teaspoon salt
- ¼ teaspoon ground black pepper
- ½ cup canned black beans, rinsed and drained
- ¼ cup diced tomatoes
- ¼ cup diced red onion
- ¼ cup crumbled feta cheese
- Two (2) tablespoons chopped fresh herbs (such as parsley, basil, or thyme)

Instructions:

1. Preheat the oven to 400°F (200°C).

2. The sweet potatoes should be sliced and put on a baking sheet.

3. Brush the sweet potatoes with the olive oil and season with the salt and pepper.

4. Bake for 15-20 minutes, or until the sweet potatoes are tender.

5. Top each sweet potato slice with the black beans, tomatoes, red onion, feta cheese, and herbs.

6. Bake for another five minutes, or until the cheese is melted.

7. Serve immediately.

8. Smoothie Bowl

Ingredients:
- 1 banana, frozen
- ½ cup frozen berries
- ½ cup plain Greek yogurt
- ¼ cup almond milk
- 2 tablespoons chia seeds
- 2 tablespoons chopped nuts (such as almonds, walnuts, or pecans)
- 2 tablespoons shredded coconut
- 2 tablespoons fresh fruit (such as strawberries, blueberries, or blackberries)

Instructions:

1. Place the banana, berries, Greek yogurt, almond milk, and chia seeds in a blender and blend until smooth.

2. Pour the smoothie into a bowl.

3. Top the smoothie with the nuts, coconut, and fresh fruit.

4. Serve immediately.

9. Breakfast Tacos

Ingredients:

- 4 whole wheat tortillas
- 4 eggs
- ½ cup skim milk
- ¼ teaspoon salt
- ¼ teaspoon ground black pepper
- ½ cup cooked, shredded chicken
- ½ cup diced bell peppers
- ½ cup diced tomatoes
- ¼ cup diced red onion
- 2 tablespoons chopped herbs (Very fresh such as parsley, basil, or thyme)
- 2 tablespoons olive oil

- ¼ cup grated cheese

Instructions:

1. A large skillet should be heated over medium heat.
2. Whisk eggs, milk, salt, and pepper together in a bowl.
3. Olive oil should be added to the skillet.
4. Add the chicken, bell peppers, tomatoes, onion, and herbs and cook for 5 minutes, stirring occasionally.
5. Pour the egg mixture into the skillet and cook for 5 minutes, stirring occasionally.
6. Divide the egg mixture among the 4 tortillas and top with the grated cheese.
7. Roll up the tortillas and serve.

10. Baked Oatmeal

Ingredients:

- 2 cups rolled oats
- 1 teaspoon baking powder
- ½ teaspoon ground cinnamon
- ½ teaspoon salt
- 2 eggs
- ½ cup skim milk
- ¼ cup honey

- 2 tablespoons olive oil
- ½ cup diced apples
- ½ cup diced pears
- ¼ cup chopped walnuts

Instructions:

1. Preheat the oven to 350°F (175°C) and lightly grease an 8-inch (20 cm) square baking dish with non-stick cooking spray.
2. In a large bowl, whisk together the oats, baking powder, cinnamon, and salt.
3. In a separate bowl, mix together the eggs, milk, honey, and olive oil.
4. The wet ingredients should be added to the dry ingredients and stir until just combined.
5. Gently fold in the apples, pears, and walnuts.
6. Spread the oatmeal mixture evenly in the baking dish.
7. Bake for 25-30 minutes, or until the oatmeal is golden brown and a toothpick inserted into the center comes out clean.
8. Allow it to cool for 10 minutes, then serve.

Chapter 3

Lunchtime Bliss: Delicious and Nutritious Recipes to Fuel Your Day

1. Sweet Potato and Black Bean Burrito Bowl

Ingredients:

- 2 tablespoons olive oil
- 1 large sweet potato, diced
- 1 cup cooked black beans
- 1 cup cooked quinoa
- 1/2 cup diced red onion
- 1/2 cup diced bell pepper
- 1/4 cup diced tomatoes
- 1 teaspoon cumin
- 1 teaspoon chili powder
- Salt and pepper to taste

Instructions:

- In a large skillet over medium-high heat, warm the olive oil.

- Add the sweet potato and cook until tender and lightly browned, about 10 minutes.
- Add the black beans, quinoa, red onion, bell pepper, tomatoes, cumin, chili powder, and salt and pepper. Cook for an additional 5 minutes.
- Serve with chosen toppings in separate bowls.

2. Mediterranean Quinoa Salad

Ingredients:
- 2 cups cooked quinoa
- 1/2 cup diced tomatoes
- 1/2 cup diced cucumber
- 1/3 cup pitted Kalamata olives
- 1/4 cup crumbled feta cheese
- 2 tablespoons olive oil
- 1 tablespoon red wine vinegar
- 1 teaspoon fresh oregano
- Salt and pepper to taste

Instructions:
- In a large bowl, combine the quinoa, tomatoes, cucumber, olives, feta cheese, olive oil, red wine vinegar, and oregano.
- Season with salt and pepper, to taste.

- Serve chilled or at room temperature.

3. Roasted Vegetable and Chickpea Bowl

Ingredients:

- 2 tablespoons olive oil
- 1 cup cubed butternut squash
- 1 cup diced zucchini
- 1 cup cooked chickpeas
- 1/2 cup diced red onion
- 1/2 cup diced bell pepper
- 1 teaspoon garlic powder
- 1 teaspoon smoked paprika
- Salt and pepper to taste

Instructions:

- Preheat oven to 400°F.
- Use parchment paper to line a baking sheet.
- In a large bowl, combine the olive oil, butternut squash, zucchini, chickpeas, red onion, bell pepper, garlic powder, smoked paprika, and salt and pepper.
- Toss to coat the vegetables.
- Spread the vegetables out on the baking sheet and roast for 20 minutes, stirring once halfway through.

- Serve in individual bowls.

4. Spinach and Artichoke Stuffed Portobello Mushrooms

Ingredients:
- 4 large portobello mushrooms
- 2 tablespoons olive oil
- 1/2 cup diced onion
- 1/2 cup diced bell pepper
- 1/4 cup diced artichokes
- 2 cups fresh baby spinach
- 1/2 cup crumbled feta cheese
- 1/4 cup grated Parmesan cheese
- Salt and pepper to taste

Instructions:
- Preheat the oven to 400°F.
- Use parchment paper to cover a baking sheet.
- Remove the stems from the Portobello mushrooms and scoop out the gills.
- In a large pot or skillet, and over medium-high heat, heat the olive oil.

- Add the onion and bell pepper and cook until softened, about five minutes.

- Add the artichokes and spinach and cook until the spinach is wilted, about 2 minutes.

- Remove the skillet from the heat and stir in the feta cheese, Parmesan cheese, and salt and pepper.

- Fill each mushroom cap with the vegetable mixture and arrange them on the baking sheet.

- Bake for 15 minutes, or until the mushrooms are tender and the cheese is melted.

5. Curried Cauliflower Rice Bowl

Ingredients:

- 2 tablespoons olive oil
- 1 head cauliflower, grated
- 1/2 cup diced onion
- 1 teaspoon curry powder
- 1/2 teaspoon ground cumin
- 1/4 teaspoon ground ginger
- 1/4 teaspoon garlic powder
- Salt and pepper to taste

Instructions:

- Heat the olive oil in a large skillet over medium-high heat.
- Add the cauliflower, onion, curry powder, cumin, ginger, garlic powder, and salt and pepper.
- Simmer for about 10 minutes, stirring periodically, or until the cauliflower is soft.
- Serve in individual bowls.

6. Cucumber and Avocado Salad

Ingredients:
- 2 large cucumbers, diced
- 2 avocados, diced
- 1/4 cup diced red onion
- 1/4 cup diced tomatoes
- 2 tablespoons olive oil
- 2 tablespoons fresh lime juice
- 1 teaspoon honey
- Salt and pepper to taste

Instructions:
- In a large bowl, combine the cucumbers, avocados, red onion, and tomatoes.
- In a small bowl, whisk together the olive oil, lime juice, honey, and salt and pepper.

- Pour the dressing over the salad and toss to coat.
- Serve chilled.

7. Baked Tofu and Vegetable Skewers

Ingredients:

- 2 tablespoons olive oil
- 1 block extra-firm tofu, drained and cubed
- 1/2 cup diced bell pepper
- 1/2 cup diced red onion
- 1/2 cup diced zucchini
- 1/4 cup diced mushrooms
- 1 teaspoon garlic powder
- 1 teaspoon smoked paprika
- Salt and pepper to taste

Instructions:

- Preheat the oven to 375°F.
- Use parchment paper to line a baking sheet.
- In a large bowl, combine the olive oil, tofu, bell pepper, red onion, zucchini, mushrooms, garlic powder, smoked paprika, and salt and pepper.
- Toss to coat the vegetables.

- Thread the vegetables and tofu onto skewers and arrange them on the baking sheet.
- Bake for 20 minutes, flipping the skewers once halfway through.

8. Mediterranean Chickpea Salad

Ingredients:

- 2 cups cooked chickpeas
- 1/2 cup diced tomatoes
- 1/2 cup diced cucumber
- 1/3 cup pitted Kalamata olives
- 1/4 cup crumbled feta cheese
- 2 tablespoons olive oil
- 1 tablespoon red wine vinegar
- 1 teaspoon fresh oregano
- Salt and pepper to taste

Instructions:

- In a large bowl, combine the chickpeas, tomatoes, cucumber, olives, feta cheese, olive oil, red wine vinegar, and oregano.
- Season with salt and pepper, to taste.
- Serve chilled or at room temperature.

9. Mediterranean Farro Bowls

Ingredients:

- 2 tablespoons olive oil
- 1 cup cooked farro
- 1/4 cup diced red onion
- 1/4 cup diced bell pepper
- 1/4 cup diced tomatoes
- 1/4 cup pitted Kalamata olives
- 1/4 cup crumbled feta cheese
- 1 teaspoon garlic powder
- 1 teaspoon dried oregano
- Salt and pepper to taste

Instructions:

- Heat the olive oil in a large skillet or pot over medium to high heat.
- Add the farro, red onion, bell pepper, tomatoes, olives, feta cheese, garlic powder, oregano, and salt and pepper.
- Cook, stirring occasionally, until the vegetables are softened. This should take about five minutes.
- Serve in individual bowls.

10. Asian Noodle Bowls

Ingredients:

- 2 tablespoons sesame oil
- 8 ounces soba noodles
- 1 cup diced mushrooms
- 1 cup diced bell pepper
- 1/2 cup diced red onion
- 2 cloves garlic, minced
- 2 tablespoons soy sauce
- 2 tablespoons rice vinegar
- 1 teaspoon grated ginger
- 1 teaspoon sesame seeds
- Salt and pepper to taste

Instructions:

- Large saucepan of salted water should be brought to a boil.
- Add the soba noodles and cook until al dente, about 8 minutes.
- Rinse the noodles in cold water after draining.

- Heat the sesame oil in a large skillet over medium-high heat.
- Add the mushrooms, bell pepper, red onion, and garlic and cook until softened, about 5 minutes.
- Add the cooked noodles, soy sauce, rice vinegar, ginger, sesame seeds, and salt and pepper.
- Cook, stirring occasionally, for an additional three minutes.
- Serve in individual bowls.

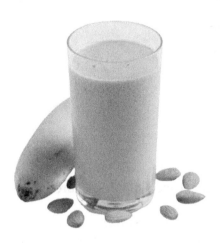

Chapter 4

Nourishing Plates: Delicious Dinners for Breast Health

1. Mediterranean Salmon with Spinach:

Ingredients:

- 4 6-ounce salmon fillets
- 2 tablespoons olive oil
- 2 cloves garlic, minced
- 2 cups fresh spinach
- ½ teaspoon sea salt
- ¼ teaspoon ground black pepper
- 2 tablespoons lemon juice
- 2 tablespoons freshly chopped parsley

Instructions:

Instructions:

1. Set the oven to 375 degrees Fahrenheit (190 degrees C).

2. Salmon filets should be placed in a baking dish.

3. Pour olive oil over the fish and season with salt, pepper, and garlic.

4. Bake the salmon for 20 minutes, or until it is done.

5. Meanwhile, heat the remaining olive oil in a large skillet over medium heat.

6. Add the spinach and cook until wilted, about 5 minutes.

7. Add the lemon juice and parsley and stir to combine.

8. Serve the salmon over the spinach.

2. Roasted Asparagus with Mushrooms:

Ingredients:
- 1 pound asparagus, trimmed
- 8 ounces mushrooms, sliced
- 2 tablespoons olive oil
- 1 teaspoon garlic powder
- ½ teaspoon sea salt
- ¼ teaspoon black pepper

Instructions:

1. Preheat the oven to 400 degrees F (approximately 200 degrees C).

2. Place asparagus and mushrooms on a baking sheet.

3. Drizzle with olive oil and sprinkle with salt, garlic powder, and pepper.

4. Roast for 15 minutes, or until the vegetables are tender.

3. Baked Sweet Potato Fries:

Ingredients:

- 2 large sweet potatoes. They should be peeled and cut into wedges
- 2 tablespoons olive oil
- ½ teaspoon garlic powder
- ½ teaspoon sea salt
- ¼ teaspoon black pepper

Instructions:

1. Preheat oven to 450 degrees F (230 degrees C).

2. Place sweet potato wedges on a baking sheet.

3. Drizzle with olive oil and sprinkle with garlic powder, salt, and pepper.

4. Bake for 20 minutes, or until the potatoes are golden and crisp.

4. Grilled Chicken with Avocado Salsa:

Ingredients:
- 4 6-ounce chicken breasts
- 2 tablespoons olive oil
- 2 teaspoons chili powder
- 1 teaspoon garlic powder
- ½ teaspoon sea salt
- ¼ teaspoon black pepper
- 1 avocado, diced
- ½ cup diced tomatoes
- ¼ cup diced red onion
- 2 tablespoons freshly chopped cilantro
- 2 tablespoons lime juice

Instructions:

1. Preheat grill to medium-high heat.
2. Brush chicken breasts with olive oil and sprinkle with chili powder, garlic powder, salt, and pepper.
3. Grill for 10 minutes, or until the chicken is cooked through.
4. Meanwhile, combine the avocado, tomatoes, red onion, cilantro, and lime juice in a bowl.
5. Serve the chicken with the avocado salsa.

5. Grilled Zucchini and Squash:

Ingredients:
- 2 medium zucchinis, sliced
- 2 medium yellow squash, sliced
- 2 tablespoons olive oil
- ½ teaspoon garlic powder
- ½ teaspoon sea salt
- ¼ teaspoon black pepper

Instructions:
1. Preheat the grill to medium-high heat.
2. Brush zucchini and squash slices with olive oil and sprinkle with garlic powder, salt, and pepper.
3. Grill for 5 minutes per side, or until the vegetables are tender and lightly charred.

6. Roasted Brussels Sprouts and Butternut Squash:

Ingredients:
- 2 cups Brussels sprouts, trimmed and halved
- 2 cups diced butternut squash
- 2 tablespoons olive oil
- ½ teaspoon garlic powder

- ½ teaspoon sea salt
- ¼ teaspoon black pepper

Instructions:

1. Set the oven to 400 degrees Fahrenheit (200 degrees C).
2. Place Brussels sprouts and butternut squash on a baking sheet.
3. Add a drizzle of olive oil and season with salt, pepper, and garlic powder.
4. Roast for 25 minutes, or until the vegetables are tender and lightly browned.

7. Quinoa and Kale Salad:

Ingredients:

- 1 cup quinoa
- 2 cups kale, chopped
- 2 tablespoons olive oil
- 2 cloves garlic, minced
- ½ teaspoon sea salt
- ¼ teaspoon black pepper
- 2 tablespoons lemon juice
- 2 tablespoons freshly chopped parsley

Instructions:

1. Cook quinoa according to package instructions.
2. Over medium heat, warm up the olive oil in a big skillet.
3. Add the kale and garlic and cook until the kale is wilted, about 5 minutes.
4. Season with some pepper and salt and remove from heat.
5. In a large bowl, combine the cooked quinoa, kale mixture, lemon juice, and parsley.
6. Serve warm or cold.

8. Grilled Portobello Mushrooms:

Ingredients:
- 4 large Portobello mushrooms, stems removed
- 2 tablespoons olive oil
- ½ teaspoon garlic powder
- ½ teaspoon sea salt
- ¼ teaspoon black pepper

Instructions:
1. Preheat the grill to medium-high heat.
2. Brush mushrooms with olive oil and sprinkle with garlic powder, salt, and pepper.
3. Grill for 5 minutes per side, or until the mushrooms are tender and lightly charred.

9. Roasted Broccoli and Cauliflower:

Ingredients:
- 2 cups broccoli florets
- 2 cups cauliflower florets
- 2 tablespoons olive oil
- ½ teaspoon garlic powder
- ½ teaspoon sea salt
- ¼ teaspoon black pepper

Instructions:

1. Preheat oven to 400 degrees F (200 degrees C).
2. Place broccoli and cauliflower florets on a baking sheet.
3. Drizzle with olive oil and sprinkle with garlic powder, salt, and pepper.
4. Roast for 20 minutes, or until the vegetables are tender and lightly browned.

10. Grilled Vegetable Skewers:

Ingredients:
- 2 bell peppers, cut into 1-inch pieces
- 2 zucchinis, cut into 1-inch pieces
- Cut 2 yellow squashes into 1-inch slices.
- 2 tablespoons olive oil

- ½ teaspoon garlic powder
- ½ teaspoon sea salt
- ¼ teaspoon black pepper

Instructions:

1. Preheat the grill to medium-high heat.
2. Thread bell peppers, zucchini, and squash onto skewers.
3. Brush with olive oil and sprinkle with garlic powder, salt, and pepper.
4. Grill for 10 minutes, or until the vegetables are tender and lightly charred.

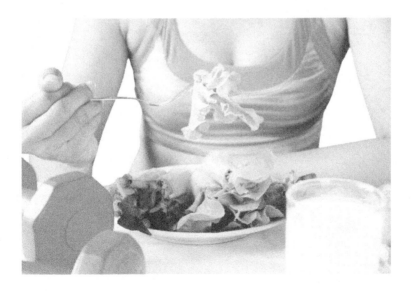

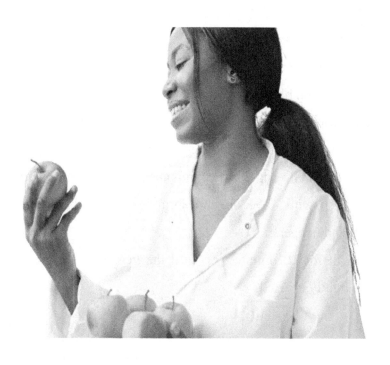

Chapter 5

Bites of Strength: Snacks & Appetizers to Empower Breast Cancer Warriors

1. Roasted Asparagus with Parmesan

Ingredients:
- 1 lb. asparagus spears
- 2 tsp. extra-virgin olive oil
- 2 Tbsp. freshly grated Parmesan

Instructions:
1. Preheat oven to 400°F.
2. Wash asparagus spears and pat dry.
3. Arrange spears in a single layer on a baking sheet.
4. Drizzle with olive oil and sprinkle with Parmesan cheese.
5. Roast for 10-12 minutes, until spears are lightly browned and tender.

2. Avocado Toast

Ingredients:
- 2 slices whole grain bread

- 1 ripe avocado
- ¼ tsp. sea salt
- Juice of ½ lemon

Instructions:

1. Toast bread slices until lightly golden.
2. Halve the avocado, scoop out the flesh, and discard the pit.
3. Mash with a fork and spread onto toast slices.
4. Sprinkle with sea salt and a squeeze of lemon juice.

3. Baked Sweet Potato Fries

Ingredients:

- 2 large sweet potatoes, peeled and cut into strips
- 2 Tbsp. extra-virgin olive oil
- ½ tsp. sea salt
- ¼ tsp. black pepper

Instructions:

1. Preheat oven to 425°F.
2. Place sweet potato strips on a baking sheet and drizzle with olive oil.
3. Sprinkle it with sea salt and pepper.

4. Bake for 20-25 minutes, flipping once halfway through, until golden and crispy.

4. Veggie Quesadillas

Ingredients:
- 2 whole wheat tortillas
- ½ cup cooked black beans
- ½ cup shredded cheese
- ½ cup chopped bell pepper
- ½ cup chopped onion
- 2 tsp. extra-virgin olive oil

Instructions:
1. Heat a nonstick skillet over medium-high heat.
2. Place one tortilla in the skillet and top with beans, cheese, bell pepper and onion.
3. Drizzle with olive oil.
4. Place the second tortilla on top and cook for 2-3 minutes, until golden and cheese is melted.
5. Flip and cook for another 2 to 3 minutes.

5. Hummus and Veggie Platter

Ingredients:
- 2 cups cooked chickpeas
- 2 cloves garlic, minced
- Juice of 1 lemon
- 2 Tbsp. tahini
- ¼ tsp. sea salt
- ½ cup diced cucumber
- ½ cup diced bell pepper
- ½ cup diced tomatoes
- ½ cup sliced olives

Instructions:

1. Place chickpeas, garlic, lemon juice, tahini and salt in a food processor and blend until smooth.
2. Arrange cucumber, bell pepper, tomatoes and olives on a platter.
3. Serve hummus with vegetables for dipping.

6. Baked Zucchini Fritters

Ingredients:
- 2 cups grated zucchini

- ½ cup whole wheat flour
- ½ cup grated Parmesan cheese
- 2 eggs, beaten
- 1 tsp. garlic powder
- ½ tsp. sea salt

Instructions:

1. Preheat oven to 375°F.
2. Squeeze water out of the zucchini with a paper towel.
3. In a medium bowl, combine zucchini, flour, Parmesan, eggs, garlic powder and salt.
4. Form into small patties and place on a parchment lined baking sheet.
5. Bake for 25 minutes, flipping halfway through, until golden and crispy.

7. Mediterranean Tuna Salad

Ingredients:

- 2 cans tuna, drained
- ½ cup diced red onion
- 1 cucumber, diced
- ½ cup diced tomatoes
- ½ cup crumbled feta cheese

- 2 Tbsp. chopped fresh parsley
- 2 Tbsp. red wine vinegar
- 2 Tbsp. extra-virgin olive oil

Instructions:

1. In a large bowl, combine tuna, onion, cucumber, tomatoes, feta cheese and parsley.
2. Combine red wine vinegar and olive oil in a small basin.
3. Pour dressing over tuna mixture and stir to combine.

8. Mediterranean Yogurt Dip

Ingredients:

- 1 cup plain Greek yogurt
- 1 clove garlic, minced
- Juice of 1 lemon
- 2 Tbsp. chopped fresh parsley
- 1 tsp. dried oregano
- ¼ tsp. sea salt
- ¼ tsp. black pepper

Instructions:

1. In a medium bowl, combine yogurt, garlic, lemon juice, parsley, oregano, salt and pepper.
2. Stir until combined.

3. It should be served with pita chips or raw vegetables.

9. Broiled Salmon with Garlic and Herbs

Ingredients:
- 2 salmon fillets
- 2 Tbsp. extra-virgin olive oil
- 2 cloves garlic, minced
- 2 Tbsp. chopped fresh parsley
- 2 Tbsp. chopped fresh dill
- 1 tsp. sea salt
- 1 tsp. black pepper

Instructions:

1. Preheat broiler to high heat.

2. Set salmon fillets on a baking pan covered with parchment paper.

3. Drizzle with olive oil and season with garlic, parsley, dill, salt and pepper.

4. Broil for 10 minutes, until cooked through and lightly browned.

10. Roasted Brussels Sprouts

Ingredients:
- 2 lb. Brussels sprouts, halved
- 2 Tbsp. extra-virgin olive oil
- ¼ tsp. sea salt
- ¼ tsp. black pepper

Instructions:

1. Preheat oven to 425°F.

2. Place Brussels sprouts on a baking sheet and drizzle with olive oil.

3. Sprinkle with salt and pepper.

4. Roast for 25-30 minutes, until lightly browned and tender.

Chapter 6

Desserts & Treats for Hope: Scrumptious Sweets to Uplift and Inspire Newly Diagnosed Breast Cancer Warriors

1. Apple and Cinnamon Oatmeal Crumble Bars

Ingredients:

- 2 cups old-fashioned oats
- 1/4 teaspoon ground cinnamon
- 1/2 teaspoon baking powder
- 1/4 teaspoon baking soda
- 1/4 teaspoon salt
- 1/2 cup melted coconut oil
- 1/2 cup coconut sugar
- 1 teaspoon pure vanilla extract
- 1/2 cup almond flour
- 1 cup diced apple
- 1/4 cup chopped walnuts

Instructions:

1. Preheat the oven to 350°F. Put parchment paper in an 8x8-inch baking pan and set it aside.
2. In a medium bowl, combine oats, cinnamon, baking powder, baking soda and salt.
3. In a separate bowl, whisk together melted coconut oil, coconut sugar and vanilla extract.
4. Stir in almond flour until combined.
5. The dry ingredients should be added to the wet ingredients and stir until combined.
6. Fold in diced apples and walnuts.
7. Spread the mixture evenly into the prepared baking pan.
8. Bake for 25-30 minutes, or until the top is golden brown and the edges are slightly crisp.
9. Allow to cool before slicing into bars.

2. Coconut Chia Seed Pudding

Ingredients:
- 1 can full-fat coconut milk
- 1/4 cup chia seeds
- 1 tablespoon maple syrup
- 1/2 teaspoon pure vanilla extract
- 1/4 teaspoon ground cinnamon

- 1/4 cup chopped walnuts

Instructions:

1. In a medium bowl, whisk together coconut milk, chia seeds, maple syrup, vanilla extract and ground cinnamon.
2. Cover and let sit in the refrigerator for at least 2 hours or overnight.
3. Stir in chopped walnuts.
4. Serve chilled in individual bowls.

3. Sweet Potato Brownies

Ingredients:

- 2 cups mashed sweet potatoes
- 1/2 cup almond butter
- 1/2 cup cocoa powder
- 1/2 cup coconut sugar
- 1 teaspoon baking powder
- 1/4 teaspoon salt
- 1 teaspoon pure vanilla extract
- 1/2 cup dark chocolate chips

Instructions:

1. Preheat oven to 350°F. Using parchment paper, line an 8x8-inch baking sheet.
2. In a medium bowl, combine mashed sweet potatoes, almond butter, cocoa powder, coconut sugar, baking powder, salt and vanilla extract.
3. Add the dark chocolate chips and mix well.
4. Spread the mixture evenly into the prepared baking pan.
5. Bake for 25-30 minutes, or until a toothpick inserted into the center comes out clean.
6. Allow to cool before slicing into brownies.

4. Banana Oat Cookies

Ingredients:
- 2 ripe bananas
- 1/2 cup almond butter
- 1/4 cup coconut sugar
- 1 teaspoon pure vanilla extract
- 2 cups old-fashioned oats
- 1/4 teaspoon baking powder
- 1/4 teaspoon baking soda
- 1/4 teaspoon salt
- 1/4 cup chopped walnuts

Instructions:

1. Preheat oven to 350°F. Put parchment paper on a baking pan and set it aside..
2. In a medium bowl, mash bananas until smooth.
3. Add almond butter, coconut sugar and vanilla extract and stir until combined.
4. Stir in oats, baking powder, baking soda and salt until combined.
5. Fold in chopped walnuts.
6. Drop the dough by rounded tablespoons onto the prepared baking sheet.
7. Bake for 12 to 15 minutes, or until the sides are just starting to brown.
8. Allow to cool before serving.

5. Raspberry Coconut Chia Popsicles

Ingredients:

- 1/2 cup chia seeds
- 1 can full-fat coconut milk
- 1/4 cup pure maple syrup
- 1 teaspoon pure vanilla extract
- 2 cups fresh raspberries

Instructions:

1. In a medium bowl, whisk together chia seeds, coconut milk, maple syrup and vanilla extract.

2. Set aside for 10 minutes to allow the mixture to thicken.

3. In a separate bowl, mash raspberries with a fork.

4. Divide the raspberry mixture among popsicle molds, filling each mold about halfway.

5. Pour the chia seed mixture over the raspberry mixture.

6. Place in the freezer for at least 4 hours, or until completely frozen.

7. Enjoy!

6. Chocolate Coconut Macaroons

Ingredients:

- 2 cups unsweetened shredded coconut
- 1/4 cup cocoa powder
- 1/4 teaspoon salt
- 1/4 cup melted coconut oil
- 1/4 cup pure maple syrup
- 1 teaspoon pure vanilla extract

Instructions:

1. Preheat oven to 350°F. Line a baking sheet with parchment paper and set aside.

2. In a medium bowl, combine shredded coconut, cocoa powder and salt.

3. Combine melted coconut oil, maple syrup, and vanilla extract in a another bowl.

4. After combining the dry ingredients, add the wet components.

5. Drop the dough by rounded tablespoons onto the prepared baking sheet.

6. Bake for 12-15 minutes, or until golden brown.

7. Allow to cool before serving.

7. Baked Apples with Walnuts and Raisins

Ingredients:
- 4 apples
- 1/2 cup chopped walnuts
- 1/4 cup raisins
- 1/4 teaspoon ground cinnamon
- 2 tablespoons melted coconut oil

Instructions:

1. Preheat oven to 350°F. A baking dish should be greased and set aside.
2. Cut the apples in half and core.
3. Place the apples cut side up in the baking dish.
4. Sprinkle with walnuts, raisins and cinnamon.
5. Drizzle with melted coconut oil.
6. Bake for 25-30 minutes, or until the apples are tender.
7. Allow to cool before serving.

8. Pear Crisp

Ingredients:

- 3 pears, peeled and diced
- 1/4 cup coconut sugar
- 1 teaspoon ground cinnamon
- 1/4 teaspoon ground nutmeg
- 1/4 teaspoon ground ginger
- 1 cup old-fashioned oats
- 1/4 cup almond flour
- 1/4 cup melted coconut oil
- 1/4 cup chopped walnuts

Instructions:

1. Preheat oven to 350°F. Grease an 8x8-inch baking dish and set aside.
2. In a medium bowl, combine pears, coconut sugar, cinnamon, nutmeg and ginger.
3. Pour the mixture into the prepared baking dish.
4. In a separate bowl, combine oats, almond flour and melted coconut oil.
5. Sprinkle the oat mixture over the pear mixture.
6. Top with chopped walnuts.
7. Bake for 25-30 minutes, or until the top is golden brown and the pears are tender.
8. Allow to cool before serving.

9. Blueberry Coconut Oat Bars

Ingredients:
- 2 cups old-fashioned oats
- 1/4 teaspoon baking powder
- 1/4 teaspoon baking soda
- 1/4 teaspoon salt
- 1/2 cup melted coconut oil
- 1/2 cup coconut sugar
- 1 teaspoon pure vanilla extract

- 1/2 cup almond flour
- 1 cup fresh blueberries
- 1/4 cup chopped walnuts

Instructions:

1. Preheat oven to 350°F. Put parchment paper in an 8x8-inch baking pan and set it aside.

2. In a medium bowl, combine oats, baking powder, baking soda and salt.

3. In a separate bowl, whisk together melted coconut oil, coconut sugar and vanilla extract.

4. Stir in almond flour until combined.

5. Add the dry ingredients to the wet ingredients and stir until combined.

6. Fold in blueberries and walnuts.

7. Spread the mixture evenly into the prepared baking pan.

8. Bake for 25-30 minutes, or until the top is golden brown and the edges are slightly crisp.

9. Allow to cool before slicing into bars.

10. No-Bake Coconut Date Balls

Ingredients:

- 2 cups pitted dates

- 1/2 cup shredded coconut
- 1/4 cup chopped walnuts
- 1 teaspoon pure vanilla extract
- 1/4 teaspoon ground cinnamon

Instructions:

1. In a food processor, combine dates, shredded coconut, walnuts, vanilla extract and cinnamon.
2. Pulse until the mixture is well combined and has a dough-like consistency.
3. Roll the dough into 1-inch balls and place them on a tray.
4. Place in the refrigerator for at least 1 hour.
5. Enjoy!

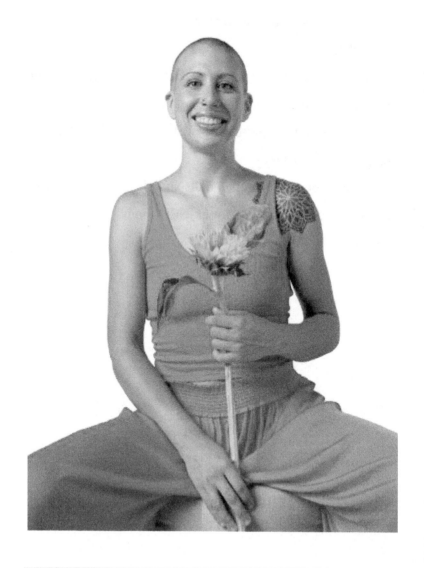

Chapter 7

Pink Blends: Delicious Juice & Smoothie Recipes for a Healthy Journey

1. Strawberry Banana Smoothie

Ingredients:
- 1 cup frozen strawberries
- 1 banana
- 1 cup low-fat, plain Greek yogurt
- 1/2 cup unsweetened almond milk
- 1/4 teaspoon ground cinnamon

Instructions:
1. All ingredients should be added to a blender and blend until smooth.
2. Serve and enjoy!

2. Green Protein Smoothie

Ingredients:
- 1 banana

- 1/2 cup spinach
- 1/2 cup frozen mango
- 1/2 cup unsweetened almond milk
- 1 scoop plant-based protein powder

Instructions:

1. Ingredients should be added to a blender and blend until smooth.
2. Serve and enjoy!

3. Pineapple Coconut Smoothie

Ingredients:

- 1 cup pineapple
- 1 banana
- 1/2 cup unsweetened almond milk
- 1/2 cup coconut cream
- 1/2 teaspoon ground turmeric

Instructions:

1. Add all ingredients to a blender and blend until smooth.
2. Serve and enjoy!

4. Carrot Apple Smoothie

Ingredients:
- 1 cup carrot juice
- 1 apple, cored and chopped
- 1/2 cup plain, unsweetened Greek yogurt
- 1/2 cup unsweetened almond milk
- 1 tablespoon ground flaxseed

Instructions:

1. After adding all ingredients to a blender, blend them until smooth.
2. Serve and enjoy!

5. Green Detox Smoothie

Ingredients:
- 1 cup spinach
- 1 banana
- 1/2 cup frozen pineapple
- 1/2 cup unsweetened almond milk
- 1 tablespoon chia seeds

Instructions:

1. Add all ingredients to a blender, then blend them until they are smooth.
2. Serve and enjoy!

6. Beet Citrus Smoothie

Ingredients:
- 1/2 cup beet juice
- 1 orange, peeled and segmented
- 1/2 cup low-fat, plain Greek yogurt
- 1/2 cup unsweetened almond milk
- 1 teaspoon ground ginger

Instructions:
1. Pour all ingredients into a blender and blend until smooth.
2. Serve and enjoy!

7. Carrot Orange Juice

Ingredients:
- 2 carrots, cut into chunks
- 2 oranges, peeled and segmented
- 1/2 cup water

Instructions:

1. Add all ingredients to a juicer and blend until smooth.

2. Serve and enjoy!

8. Berry Spinach Juice

Ingredients:
- 1 cup strawberries
- 1 cup spinach
- 1/2 cup water

Instructions:

1. Add all ingredients to a juicer and blend until smooth.

2. Serve and enjoy!

9. Spicy Pineapple Juice

Ingredients:
- 1 cup pineapple
- 1/2 lemon, peeled and segmented
- 1/2 teaspoon ground cayenne pepper
- 1/2 cup water

Instructions:

1. Add all ingredients to a juicer and blend until smooth.

2. Serve and enjoy!

10. Creamy Coconut Smoothie

Ingredients:
- 1 banana
- 1/2 cup coconut milk
- 1/2 cup plain, unsweetened Greek yogurt
- 1 tablespoon honey

Instructions:

1. Pour all ingredients into a blender and blend until smooth.

2. Serve and enjoy!

Chapter 8

Heartful Bowls: Veggie Recipes for Newly Diagnosed Breast Cancer Thrivers

1. Roasted Butternut Squash, Brussels sprouts, and Chickpeas:

Ingredients:
- 2 cups of cubed butternut squash
- 2 cups of Brussels sprouts, halved
- 1 cup of cooked chickpeas
- 2 tablespoons of olive oil
- 1 teaspoon of garlic powder
- 1 teaspoon of dried oregano
- ½ teaspoon of salt
- ¼ teaspoon of pepper

Instructions:
- Preheat the oven to 400°F.
- Butternut squash and brussels sprouts should be placed in a large bowl.

- Drizzle with olive oil and season with oregano, salt, garlic powder, and pepper.
- Toss to evenly coat.
- Vegetables should be spread onto a baking sheet.
- Bake for 20-25 minutes, or until the vegetables are softened and lightly browned.
- Add cooked chickpeas to the baking sheet during the last 5 minutes of baking.
- Serve warm in a bowl.

2. Zucchini Noodle Salad with Avocado:

Ingredients:
- 2 large zucchini, spiralizer into noodles
- 1 ripe avocado, diced
- 1 cup of cherry tomatoes, halved
- ½ cup of freshly chopped cilantro
- 2 tablespoons of olive oil
- 1 tablespoon of lime juice
- 1 teaspoon of garlic powder
- ¼ teaspoon of salt
- ¼ teaspoon of pepper

Instructions:

- Zucchini noodles should be put in a large bowl.
- Add avocado, cherry tomatoes, and cilantro.
- Drizzle with oil (olive) and lime juice.
- Add salt, pepper, and garlic powder for seasoning.
- Toss to evenly coat.
- Serve chilled in a bowl.

3. Roasted Sweet Potato and Red Pepper Soup:

Ingredients:
- 2 large sweet potatoes, cubed
- 1 large red pepper, diced
- 1 cup of vegetable broth
- ½ cup of canned coconut milk
- 1 tablespoon of olive oil
- 1 teaspoon of garlic powder
- 1 teaspoon of ground cumin
- ½ teaspoon of paprika
- ½ teaspoon of salt

Instructions:
- Preheat the oven to 400°F.
- Place sweet potatoes and red pepper on a baking sheet.

- Drizzle with olive oil and season with garlic powder, cumin, paprika, and salt.
- Toss to evenly coat.
- Roast for 20-25 minutes, or until the vegetables are tender.
- Roasted vegetables should be transferred to a blender.
- Add vegetable broth and coconut milk.
- Blend until smooth and creamy.
- Serve warm in a bowl.

4. Quinoa and Kale Power Bowl:

Ingredients:
- 2 cups of cooked quinoa
- 2 cups of chopped kale
- ½ cup of cooked chickpeas
- ½ cup of diced red onion
- ¼ cup of freshly chopped parsley
- 2 tablespoons of olive oil
- 1 tablespoon of lemon juice
- 1 teaspoon of garlic powder
- ½ teaspoon of salt

Instructions:

- Place quinoa, kale, chickpeas, and red onion in a large bowl.
- Drizzle with lemon juice and olive oil
- Season with garlic powder and salt.
- Toss to evenly coat.
- Top with freshly chopped parsley.
- Serve warm in a bowl.

5. Roasted Broccoli, Carrots, and Chickpeas:

Ingredients:
- 2 cups of broccoli florets
- 2 cups of sliced carrots
- 1 cup of cooked chickpeas
- 2 tablespoons of olive oil
- 1 teaspoon of garlic powder
- 1 teaspoon of ground cumin
- ½ teaspoon of salt
- ¼ teaspoon of pepper

Instructions:
- Preheat oven to 400°F.
- Place broccoli, carrots, and chickpeas in a large bowl.

- It should be drizzled with olive oil, and seasoned with cumin, garlic powder, salt, and pepper.
- Toss to evenly coat.
- On a baking sheet, spread the vegetables out evenly.
- On a baking sheet, spread the vegetables out evenly.
- Bake the vegetables for 20 to 25 minutes, or until they are soft and just beginning to brown.
- Serve warm in a bowl.

6. Spicy Black Bean and Quinoa Bowl:

Ingredients:
- 2 cups of cooked quinoa
- 1 cup of cooked black beans
- ½ cup of diced red onion
- ½ cup of diced red pepper
- ¼ cup of freshly chopped cilantro
- 2 tablespoons of olive oil
- 1 tablespoon of lime juice
- 1 teaspoon of garlic powder
- ½ teaspoon of cayenne pepper
- ½ teaspoon of salt

Instructions:

- Place quinoa, black beans, red onion, and red pepper in a large bowl.
- Drizzle with olive oil and lime juice.
- Season with garlic powder, cayenne pepper, and salt.
- Toss to evenly coat.
- Top with freshly chopped cilantro.
- Serve warm in a bowl.

7. Baked Eggplant and Chickpea Curry:

Ingredients:
- 2 large eggplants, cubed
- 1 cup of cooked chickpeas
- 1 cup of diced tomatoes
- ½ cup of diced onion
- 2 tablespoons of olive oil
- 1 tablespoon of curry powder
- 1 teaspoon of ground ginger
- ½ teaspoon of cumin
- ½ teaspoon of salt

Instructions:
- Preheat the oven to 400°F.

- Place eggplant and chickpeas in a large bowl.
- Drizzle with olive oil and season with curry powder, ginger, cumin, and salt.
- Toss to evenly coat.
- On a baking sheet, spread the vegetables.
- Bake the vegetables for 20 to 25 minutes, or until they are cooked through and slightly browned.
- Add diced tomatoes and onion during the last 5 minutes of baking.
- Serve warm in a bowl.

8. Roasted Cauliflower and Chickpea Bowl:

Ingredients:
- 2 cups of cauliflower florets
- 1 cup of cooked chickpeas
- 2 tablespoons of olive oil
- 1 teaspoon of garlic powder
- 1 teaspoon of ground cumin
- ½ teaspoon of smoked paprika
- ½ teaspoon of salt
- ¼ teaspoon of pepper

Instructions:

- Preheat oven to 400°F.
- Place cauliflower and chickpeas in a large bowl.
- Drizzle with olive oil and season with garlic powder, cumin, smoked paprika, salt, and pepper.
- Toss to evenly coat.
- Onto a baking sheet, spread the vegetables.
- Bake the vegetables for 20 to 25 minutes, or until they are soft and have a slight browned crust.
- Serve warm in a bowl.

9. Kale and Avocado Salad:

Ingredients:
- 2 cups of chopped kale
- 1 ripe avocado, diced
- ½ cup of diced red onion
- ¼ cup of freshly chopped parsley
- 2 tablespoons of olive oil
- 1 tablespoon of lemon juice
- 1 teaspoon of garlic powder
- ½ teaspoon of salt

Instructions:
- Place kale, avocado, and red onion in a large bowl.

- Drizzle with olive oil and lemon juice.
- Season with garlic powder and salt.
- Toss to evenly coat.
- Top with freshly chopped parsley.
- Serve chilled in a bowl.

10. Quinoa and Roasted Veggies Bowl:

Ingredients:
- 2 cups of cooked quinoa
- 1 cup of cubed butternut squash
- 1 cup of sliced carrots
- 1 cup of sliced bell pepper
- 2 tablespoons of olive oil
- 1 teaspoon of garlic powder
- ½ teaspoon of dried oregano
- ½ teaspoon of salt
- ¼ teaspoon of pepper

Instructions:
- Preheat the oven to 400°F.
- Place butternut squash, carrots, and bell pepper in a large bowl.

- Drizzle with olive oil and season with garlic powder, oregano, salt, and pepper.
- Toss to evenly coat.
- Arrange the vegetables on a baking sheet.
- Bake the vegetables for 20 to 25 minutes, or until they are soft and gently browned.
- Place cooked quinoa in a bowl.
- Top with roasted vegetables.
- Serve warm in a bowl.

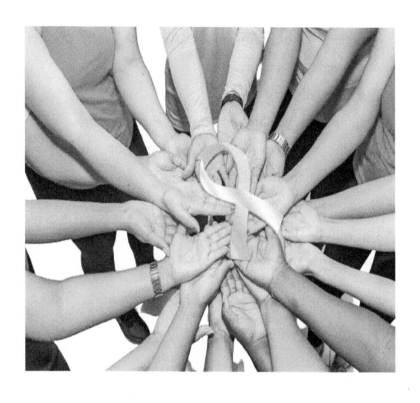

Chapter 9

Green for Hope: Delicious Salads Recipes for Newly Diagnosed Breast Cancer Fighters

1. Broccoli and Tomato Salad:

Ingredients:
- 2 cups of broccoli florets
- 1 cup of halved cherry tomatoes
- 2 tablespoons of olive oil
- A tablespoon of freshly squeezed lemon juice
- Salt and pepper to taste

Instructions:
- In a medium bowl, combine the broccoli and tomatoes.
- In a small bowl, whisk together the olive oil, lemon juice, salt and pepper.
- Pour the dressing over the vegetables and toss to coat.
- Serve the salad chilled or at room temperature.

2. Avocado and Spinach Salad:

Ingredients:
- 4 cups of fresh baby spinach
- 1 large avocado, diced
- Freshly squeezed lime juice, 2 tablespoons
- 2 tablespoons of olive oil
- Salt and pepper to taste

Instructions:
- In a large bowl, combine the spinach and avocado.
- Whisk together olive oil, salt, lime juice and pepper in a small bowl
- Douse the salad in the dressing, then toss to combine.
- Salads are best when served chilled or at room temperature.

3. Kale and Roasted Sweet Potato Salad:

Ingredients:
- 2 cups of chopped kale
- 2 cups of roasted sweet potatoes, cubed

- 2 tablespoons of olive oil
- 2 tablespoons of honey
- Salt and pepper to taste

Instructions:
- In a large bowl, combine the kale and sweet potatoes.
- In a small bowl, whisk together the olive oil, honey, salt and pepper.
- Put the dressing over the salad and toss to coat.
- Salad can be served cold or at room temperature.

4. Quinoa and Black Bean Salad:

Ingredients:
- 2 cups of cooked quinoa
- 1 cup of cooked black beans
- ½ cup of diced red pepper
- 2 tablespoons of olive oil
- Freshly squeezed lime juice, 2 tablespoon
- Salt and pepper to taste

Instructions:

- In a large bowl, combine the quinoa, black beans and red pepper.
- In a small bowl, whisk together the olive oil, lime juice, salt and pepper.
- Pour the dressing over the salad and combine to coat.
- Salad should be served chilled or at room temperature.

5. Roasted Beet and Feta Salad:

Ingredients:
- 2 cups of roasted beets, cubed
- ½ cup of crumbled feta cheese
- 2 tablespoons of olive oil
- Lemon juice, freshly squeezed, 2 tablespoons
- Salt and pepper to taste

Instructions:
- In a large bowl, combine the feta cheese and beets.
- In a small bowl, whisk together the pepper, olive oil, lemon juice and salt.
- Drizzle the salad with the dressing and toss to combine.
- Salad can be served cold or at room temperature.

6. Carrot and Chickpea Salad:

Ingredients:

- 2 cups of grated carrots
- 1 cup of cooked chickpeas
- 2 tablespoons of olive oil
- 2 tablespoons of freshly squeezed orange juice
- Salt and pepper to taste

Instructions:

- In a large bowl, combine the carrots and chickpeas.
- Combine the olive oil, honey, salt, and pepper in a small bowl.
- Pour the dressing over the salad and toss to coat.
- Salad can be served cold or at room temperature.

7. Cucumber and Tomato Salad:

Ingredients:

- 2 cups of diced cucumber
- 1 cup of halved cherry tomatoes
- 2 tablespoons of olive oil

- 2 tablespoons of freshly squeezed lemon juice
- Salt and pepper to taste

Instructions:

- In a large bowl, combine the cucumber and tomatoes.
- In a small bowl, whisk together the olive oil, lemon juice, salt and pepper.
- Put the dressing over the salad and toss to coat.
- Serve salad chilled or at room temperature.

8. Apple and Walnut Salad:

Ingredients:

- 2 cups of diced apples
- ½ cup of chopped walnuts
- 2 tablespoons of olive oil
- 2 tablespoons of honey
- Salt and pepper to taste

Instructions:

- In a large bowl, combine the apples and walnuts.
- Combine the olive oil, honey, salt, and pepper in a small bowl.

- Pour the dressing over the salad and toss to coat.
- Salad can be served at room temperature or if preferred, cold.

9. Zucchini and Feta Salad:

Ingredients:
- 2 cups of grated zucchini
- ½ cup of crumbled feta cheese
- 2 tablespoons of olive oil
- 2 tablespoons of freshly squeezed lemon juice
- Salt and pepper to taste

Instructions:
- In a large bowl, combine the zucchini and feta cheese.
- Whisk together the olive oil, lemon juice, salt and pepper in a bowl (small bowl).
- The dressing should be poured over the salad and tossed to coat.
- Serve the salad chilled, or at room temperature if preferred.

10. Quinoa and Apple Salad:

Ingredients:
- 2 cups of cooked quinoa
- 2 cups of diced apples
- 2 tablespoons of olive oil
- 2 tablespoons of honey
- Salt and pepper to taste

Instructions:
- In a large bowl, combine the quinoa and apples.
- In a bowl, whisk together the honey, olive oil, salt and pepper.
- The dressing should be poured over the salad and tossed to coat.
- Serve the salad chilled, or at room temperature if preferred.

Chapter 10

Stronger Together: Nutritious and Flavorful Sides Recipes for Fighting Breast Cancer

1. Lentil and Squash Stew with Cumin-Roasted Chickpeas

Ingredients:

- 2 tablespoons olive oil
- 1 cup chopped onion
- 2 cloves garlic, minced
- 1 teaspoon cumin
- 1 teaspoon ground coriander
- 1 teaspoon smoked paprika
- 1/2 teaspoon ground turmeric
- 1/2 teaspoon ground cinnamon
- 1/4 teaspoon cayenne pepper
- 2 cups vegetable broth
- 1/2 cup lentils, rinsed
- 1/2 cup diced carrot

- 1/2 cup diced celery
- 1 can diced tomatoes
- 1 small butternut squash, peeled and diced
- 1 can chickpeas, drained and rinsed
- 2 tablespoons olive oil
- 1 teaspoon ground cumin
- Salt and pepper, to taste

Instructions:

1. In a large pot, heat olive oil over medium heat. Add onion and garlic, and cook until softened, about 5 minutes.

2. Add cumin, coriander, smoked paprika, turmeric, cinnamon, and cayenne pepper. Cook for 1 minute, stirring constantly.

3. Add the broth, lentils, carrots, celery, tomatoes, and butternut squash. Bring the mixture to a boil, reduce heat to low, and simmer, covered, for 20 minutes.

4. Preheat oven to 425F. Line a baking sheet with parchment paper.

5. In a bowl, combine chickpeas, olive oil, cumin, salt and pepper. Toss to coat.

6. Spread chickpeas onto prepared baking sheet and roast in preheated oven for 15 minutes.

7. When stew is finished cooking, stir in roasted chickpeas. Serve warm.

2. Broccoli and Quinoa Salad

Ingredients:
- 2 cups uncooked quinoa
- 4 cups broccoli florets
- 4 tablespoons olive oil
- Juice of 1 lemon
- 2 cloves garlic, minced
- 1/4 teaspoon ground turmeric
- 1/4 teaspoon ground cumin
- 1/4 cup chopped fresh parsley
- 1/2 teaspoon salt
- 1/4 teaspoon black pepper

Instructions:
1. Cook quinoa according to package instructions.
2. In a large bowl, combine cooked quinoa and broccoli florets.
3. In a small bowl, whisk together olive oil, lemon juice, garlic, turmeric, cumin, parsley, salt and pepper.

4. Pour dressing over quinoa and broccoli and toss to combine. Serve at room temperature or chilled.

3. Kale and Roasted Beet Salad

Ingredients:

- Kale, 2 bunches leaves chopped and stems removed
- 2 large beets, peeled and diced
- 2 tablespoons olive oil
- 1 tablespoon balsamic vinegar
- 2 cloves garlic, minced
- 1/4 teaspoon ground cumin
- 1/4 teaspoon ground coriander
- 1/4 teaspoon ground turmeric
- 1/4 teaspoon salt
- 1/4 teaspoon black pepper

Instructions:

1. Preheat oven to 400F. Baking sheet should be lined with parchment paper.

2. Place diced beets onto a prepared baking sheet and drizzle with olive oil. Roast in a preheated oven for about twenty minutes.

3. In a large bowl, combine roasted beets and kale.

4. In a small bowl, whisk together balsamic vinegar, garlic, cumin, coriander, turmeric, salt, and pepper.

5. Pour dressing over kale and beets and toss to combine. Serve at room temperature or chilled.

4. Zucchini Noodle Bowl with Garlic-Miso Sauce

Ingredients:

- 2 tablespoons olive oil
- 2 cloves garlic, minced
- 2 tablespoons white miso paste
- 2 tablespoons rice vinegar
- 1 tablespoon sesame oil
- 2 tablespoons honey
- 2 large zucchinis, spiralized
- 1 cup edamame, cooked
- 1 cup shredded carrot
- 1/2 cup chopped cilantro

Instructions:

1. In a small bowl, whisk together olive oil, garlic, miso paste, rice vinegar, sesame oil, and honey.

2. In a large bowl, combine spiralized zucchini, edamame, carrots, and cilantro.

3. Pour garlic-miso sauce over zucchini noodles and toss to combine. Serve at room temperature or chilled.

5. Quinoa Cakes with Spinach and Feta

Ingredients:

- 1 cup cooked quinoa
- 1/2 cup cooked spinach
- 1/2 cup crumbled feta cheese
- 2 eggs, lightly beaten
- 1/4 cup almond flour
- 1/4 teaspoon ground cumin
- 1/4 teaspoon garlic powder
- Salt and pepper, to taste
- 2 tablespoons olive oil

Instructions:

1. In a large bowl, combine quinoa, spinach, feta cheese, eggs, almond flour, cumin, garlic powder, salt and pepper. Mix until well combined.

2. Heat olive oil in a large pot, or a skillet over medium heat.

3. Form quinoa mixture into small patties and add to preheated skillet. Cook for 2-3 minutes per side, or until golden brown.

4. Serve quinoa cakes warm.

6. Sweet Potato and Chickpea Curry

Ingredients:

- 2 tablespoons olive oil
- 1 onion, diced
- 2 cloves garlic, minced
- 1 teaspoon ground cumin
- 1 teaspoon ground coriander
- 1 teaspoon ground turmeric
- 1/2 teaspoon ground ginger
- 1/4 teaspoon cayenne pepper
- Sweet potato, large, peeled and diced
- 1 can chickpeas, drained and rinsed
- 1 can diced tomatoes
- 1 cup vegetable broth
- Salt and pepper, to taste

Instructions:

1. Olive oil should be heated in a large pot over medium heat. Also add garlic and onions, and cook until softened. This should take about 5 minutes.

2. Add cumin, coriander, turmeric, ginger, and cayenne pepper. Cook for 1 minute, stirring constantly.

3. Add sweet potato, chickpeas, tomatoes, and vegetable broth. Bring the mixture to a boil, reduce heat to low, and simmer, covered, for 20 minutes.

4. Season with salt and pepper, to taste. Serve warm.

7. Grilled Eggplant and Zucchini with Rosemary

Ingredients:

- 2 tablespoons olive oil

- 2 cloves garlic, minced

- 2 teaspoons chopped fresh rosemary

- 1/4 teaspoon ground cumin

- 1/4 teaspoon ground coriander

- 1/4 teaspoon ground turmeric

- Large eggplant, sliced into a quarter of an inch thick rounds

- 1 large zucchini, sliced into 1/4-inch thick rounds

- Salt and pepper, to taste

Instructions:

1. Heat olive oil in a large skillet over medium heat. Add garlic, rosemary, cumin, coriander, and turmeric, and cook for 1 minute.

2. Add eggplant and zucchini to the skillet and season with salt and pepper. Cook for 5-7 minutes, or until vegetables are tender.

3. Preheat the grill to high heat.

4. Grill vegetables for 2-3 minutes per side, or until lightly charred. Serve warm.

8. Roasted Cauliflower and Chickpea Bowl

Ingredients:

- Cauliflower, 1 head, cut into florets
- 4 tablespoons olive oil
- 2 cloves garlic, minced
- 1 teaspoon ground cumin
- 1 teaspoon ground coriander
- 1/2 teaspoon ground turmeric
- 1/4 teaspoon cayenne pepper
- 1 can chickpeas, drained and rinsed

- 1/2 cup diced red onion
- 1/4 cup chopped fresh parsley
- 1/4 cup crumbled feta cheese
- Salt and pepper, to taste

Instructions:

1. Preheat the oven to 425 F. Use parchment paper to line a baking sheet.
2. Place cauliflower florets onto a prepared baking sheet and drizzle with 2 tablespoons olive oil. Roast in a preheated oven for approximately about 20 minutes.
3. In a large skillet, heat remaining 2 tablespoons of olive oil over medium heat. Add garlic, cumin, coriander, turmeric, and cayenne pepper. Cook for 1 minute, stirring constantly.
4. Add chickpeas, red onion, and roasted cauliflower and cook for 5 minutes.
5. Stir in parsley and feta cheese and season with salt and pepper, to taste. Serve warm.

9. Roasted Vegetable and Couscous Bowl

Ingredients:

- 2 tablespoons olive oil

- 1 onion, diced
- 2 cloves garlic, minced
- 1 red bell pepper, diced
- 1 zucchini, diced
- 1 teaspoon ground cumin
- 1 teaspoon ground coriander
- 1/2 teaspoon ground turmeric
- 1 can diced tomatoes
- 1 cup vegetable broth
- 1 cup uncooked couscous
- 1/4 cup chopped fresh parsley
- Salt and pepper, to taste

Instructions:

1. Preheat the oven to 400F. Use parchment paper to cover a baking sheet.
2. Place onion, garlic, bell pepper, and zucchini onto a prepared baking sheet and drizzle with olive oil. Roast for 20 minutes in a preheated oven.
3. In a large saucepan, heat remaining olive oil over medium heat. Add cumin, coriander, and turmeric. Cook for 1 minute, stirring constantly.

4. Add diced tomatoes and vegetable broth and bring to a boil. Turn down the heat, cover, and simmer for ten minutes.

5. Stir in couscous and roasted vegetables. For 5 minutes, cover and leave standing.

6. Fluff with a fork and stir in parsley. Season with salt and pepper, to taste. Serve warm.

10. Roasted Carrot and Lentil Salad

Ingredients:

- 2 tablespoons olive oil
- 1 pound carrots, peeled and diced
- 2 cloves garlic, minced
- 1 teaspoon ground cumin
- 1 teaspoon ground coriander
- 1/2 teaspoon ground turmeric
- 1/2 teaspoon smoked paprika
- 1/4 cup uncooked lentils
- 2 cups vegetable broth
- Juice of 1 lemon
- 1/4 cup chopped fresh parsley
- Salt and pepper, to taste

Instructions:

1. Preheat oven to 400F. Put parchment paper on a baking pan to line it.

2. Place diced carrots onto prepared baking sheet and drizzle with olive oil. 20 minutes of roasting should be done in a preheated oven.

3. In a large saucepan, heat remaining olive oil over medium heat. Add garlic, cumin, coriander, turmeric, and smoked paprika. Cook for 1 minute, stirring constantly.

4. Add lentils, vegetable broth, and lemon juice. Bring the mixture to a boil, reduce heat to low, and simmer, covered, for 20 minutes.

5. When lentils are finished cooking, stir in roasted carrots and parsley. Season with salt and pepper, to taste. Serve warm.

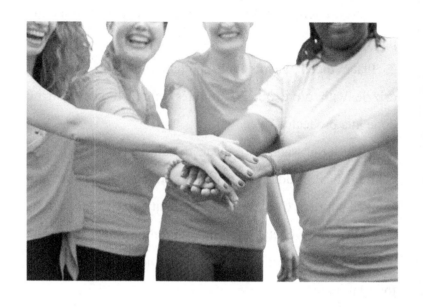

Chapter 11

Bowlfuls of Bravery: Delicious & Heartwarming Soups for Breast Health

1. Roasted Tomato and Red Pepper Soup

Ingredients:
- 4 large tomatoes, quartered
- 1 large red pepper, quartered
- 2 cloves garlic, minced
- 2 tablespoons olive oil
- 1 teaspoon ground black pepper
- 1 teaspoon dried oregano
- 1 teaspoon dried basil
- 1/2 teaspoon sea salt
- 3 cups vegetable broth

Instructions:
1. Preheat oven to 400°F.
2. Arrange tomatoes and red pepper on a baking sheet.
3. Drizzle olive oil over the vegetables and sprinkle with pepper, oregano, basil, and salt.

4. Roast in the oven for 20-25 minutes, or until vegetables are soft and lightly browned.

5. Transfer roasted vegetables to a blender and puree until smooth.

6. Transfer pureed vegetables to a large pot and add vegetable broth.

7. Simmer for 15 to 20 minutes at medium-low heat.

8. Serve and enjoy!

2. Creamy Carrot Soup

Ingredients:

- 4 large carrots, peeled and chopped
- 1 onion, chopped
- 2 cloves garlic, minced
- 2 tablespoons olive oil
- 1 teaspoon ground black pepper
- 1 teaspoon dried thyme
- 1/2 teaspoon sea salt
- 3 cups vegetable broth
- 1/4 cup nutritional yeast

Instructions:

1. In a big pot set over medium heat, warm the olive oil.

2. Add carrots, onion, and garlic to the pot and sauté for 5 minutes, or until vegetables are softened.

3. Add pepper, thyme, and salt to the pot and stir to combine.

4. Add veggie broth and heat through.

5. Reduce heat to low and simmer for 15-20 minutes, or until carrots are tender.

6. Remove soup from heat and transfer to a blender.

7. Add nutritional yeast to the blender and puree until smooth.

8. Pour soup back into the pot and simmer for an additional 10 minutes.

9. Serve and enjoy!

3. Cauliflower and Leek Soup

Ingredients:
- 1 head cauliflower, broken into florets
- 2 leeks, chopped
- 2 cloves garlic, minced
- 2 tablespoons olive oil
- 1 teaspoon ground black pepper
- 1 teaspoon dried thyme

- 1/2 teaspoon sea salt
- 3 cups vegetable broth

Instructions:

1. Olive oil should be heated in a large pot, and over medium heat.
2. Add leeks and garlic to the pot and sauté for 5 minutes, or until vegetables are softened.
3. Add cauliflower, pepper, thyme, and salt to the pot and stir to combine.
4. Add or pour in vegetable broth and bring to a boil.
5. Reduce heat to low and simmer for 15-20 minutes, or until cauliflower is tender.
6. Remove soup from heat and transfer to a blender.
7. Puree until smooth.
8. Pour soup back into the pot and simmer for an additional 10 minutes.
9. Serve and enjoy!

4. Lentil Soup

Ingredients:

- 1 cup red lentils, rinsed
- 2 carrots, peeled and chopped

- 2 stalks celery, chopped
- 2 cloves garlic, minced
- 2 tablespoons olive oil
- 1 teaspoon ground black pepper
- 1 teaspoon dried oregano
- 1/2 teaspoon sea salt
- 3 cups vegetable broth

Instructions:

1. Heat olive oil in a large pot over medium heat.
2. Add carrots, celery, and garlic to the pot and sauté for 5 minutes, or until vegetables are softened.
3. Add lentils, pepper, oregano, and salt to the pot and stir to combine.
4. Bring to a boil after adding the vegetable broth.
5. Reduce heat to low and simmer for 15-20 minutes, or until lentils are tender.
6. Remove soup from heat and adjust seasoning to taste.
7. Serve and enjoy!

5. Asparagus Soup

Ingredients:

- 1 bunch asparagus, chopped

- 1 onion, chopped
- 2 cloves garlic, minced
- 2 tablespoons olive oil
- 1 teaspoon ground black pepper
- 1 teaspoon dried oregano
- 1/2 teaspoon sea salt
- 3 cups vegetable broth

Instructions:

1. Heat olive oil in a large pot over medium heat.
2. Add onion and garlic to the pot and sauté for 5 minutes, or until vegetables are softened.
3. Add asparagus, pepper, oregano, and salt to the pot and stir to combine.
4. Vegetable broth should be added and brought to a boil.
5. Reduce heat to low and simmer for 15-20 minutes, or until asparagus is tender.
6. Remove soup from heat and transfer to a blender.
7. Puree until smooth.
8. Pour soup back into the pot and simmer for an additional 10 minutes.
9. Serve and enjoy!

6. Kale and White Bean Soup

Ingredients:
- 1 bunch kale, chopped
- White beans, rinsed and drained, 2 cans
- 1 onion, chopped
- 2 cloves garlic, minced
- 2 tablespoons olive oil
- 1 teaspoon ground black pepper
- 1 teaspoon dried thyme
- 1/2 teaspoon sea salt
- 3 cups vegetable broth

Instructions:

1. Over medium heat, warm up the olive oil in a big pot.

2. Add onion and garlic to the pot and sauté for 5 minutes, or until vegetables are softened.

3. Add kale, pepper, thyme, and salt to the pot and stir to combine.

4. Pour in white beans and vegetable broth and bring to a boil.

5. Reduce heat to low and simmer for 15-20 minutes, or until kale is tender.

6. Remove soup from heat and adjust seasoning to taste.

7. Serve and enjoy!

7. Broccoli and Cheddar Soup

Ingredients:
- 1 head broccoli, chopped
- 2 cups cheddar cheese, shredded
- 1 onion, chopped
- 2 cloves garlic, minced
- 2 tablespoons olive oil
- 1 teaspoon ground black pepper
- 1 teaspoon dried oregano
- 1/2 teaspoon sea salt
- 3 cups vegetable broth

Instructions:

1. In a big pot, warm up the olive oil over medium heat.

2. Add onion and garlic to the pot and sauté for 5 minutes, or until vegetables are softened.

3. Add broccoli, pepper, oregano, and salt to the pot and stir to combine.

4. Bring to a boil, after you've poured vegetable broth.

5. Reduce heat to low and simmer for 15-20 minutes, or until broccoli is tender.

6. Remove soup from heat and stir in cheddar cheese until melted.

7. Serve and enjoy!

8. Butternut Squash Soup

Ingredients:
- 1 large butternut squash, peeled and cubed
- 2 carrots, peeled and chopped
- 2 cloves garlic, minced
- 2 tablespoons olive oil
- 1 teaspoon ground black pepper
- 1 teaspoon dried thyme
- 1/2 teaspoon sea salt
- 3 cups vegetable broth

Instructions:

1. Heat up olive oil in a large pot, and over medium heat.

2. Add carrots and garlic to the pot and sauté for 5 minutes, or until vegetables are softened.

3. Add butternut squash, pepper, thyme, and salt to the pot and stir to combine.

4. Vegetable broth should be added and brought to a boil.

5. Reduce heat to low and simmer for 15-20 minutes, or until squash is tender.

6. Remove soup from heat and transfer to a blender.

7. Puree until smooth.

8. Pour soup back into the pot and simmer for an additional 10 minutes.

9. Serve and enjoy!

9. Parsnip and Potato Soup

Ingredients:

- 2 large parsnips, peeled and chopped
- 2 potatoes, peeled and chopped
- 1 onion, chopped
- 2 cloves garlic, minced
- 2 tablespoons olive oil
- 1 teaspoon ground black pepper
- 1 teaspoon dried oregano
- 1/2 teaspoon sea salt
- 3 cups vegetable broth

Instructions:

1. Heat olive oil in a large pot over medium heat.

2. Add onion and garlic to the pot and sauté for 5 minutes, or until vegetables are softened.

3. Add parsnips, potatoes, pepper, oregano, and salt to the pot and stir to combine.

4. Pour in vegetable broth and bring to a boil.

5. Reduce heat to low and simmer for 15-20 minutes, or until vegetables are tender.

6. Remove soup from heat and transfer to a blender.

7. Puree until smooth.

8. Pour soup back into the pot and simmer for an additional 10 minutes.

9. Serve and enjoy!

10. Sweet Potato and Cumin Soup

Ingredients:
- Two large sweet potatoes, peeled and cubed
- 1 onion, chopped
- 2 cloves garlic, minced
- 2 tablespoons olive oil
- 1 teaspoon ground cumin
- 1 teaspoon ground black pepper
- 1/2 teaspoon sea salt

- 3 cups vegetable broth

Instructions:

1. Heat olive oil in a large pot or skillet over medium heat.

2. Add onion and garlic to the pot and sauté for 5 minutes, or until vegetables are softened.

3. Add sweet potatoes, cumin, pepper, and salt to the pot and stir to combine.

4. When the broth has been added, turn the heat to high.

5. Reduce heat to low and simmer for 15-20 minutes, or until potatoes are tender.

6. Remove soup from heat and transfer to a blender.

7. Blend thoroughly.

8. Refill the pot with the soup, then cook it for 10 more minutes.

9. Serve and enjoy!

Chapter 12

30 Days Culinary Crusade for Newly Diagnosed Breast Cancer Fighters

Day 1:

Breakfast: Chia seeds with overnight oats, almond milk, and berries.

Lunch: Quinoa and black bean salad with olive oil and lemon juice.

Dinner: Baked salmon with steamed vegetables.

Snack: Apple slices with almond butter.

Day 2:

Breakfast: Egg scramble with bell peppers, onions, and spinach.

Lunch: Hummus wrap with lettuce, tomato, and cucumber.

Dinner: Baked chicken with roasted sweet potatoes and broccoli.

Snack: Greek yogurt with berries.

Day 3:

Breakfast: Avocado toast with a side of scrambled eggs.

Lunch: Lentil soup with a side of steamed vegetables.

Dinner: Baked cod with roasted cauliflower and asparagus.

Snack: Celery sticks with peanut butter.

Day 4:

Breakfast: Oatmeal with almond milk, chia seeds, and banana.

Lunch: Grilled turkey sandwich with lettuce and tomato.

Dinner: Turkey breast (roasted), with mashed potatoes and green beans.

Snack: Carrot sticks with hummus.

Day 5:

Breakfast: Greek yogurt parfait with berries and granola.

Lunch: lettuce, tomato, and cucumber with tuna salad.

Dinner: Vegetable stir fry with brown rice.

Snack: Edamame with sea salt.

Day 6:

Breakfast: Egg muffins with spinach, peppers and cheese.

Lunch: Chickpea and quinoa salad with olive oil and lemon juice.

Dinner: Baked tilapia with roasted potatoes and Brussels sprouts.

Snack: Apple slices with almond butter.

Day 7:

Breakfast: Almond milk, spinach, protein powder and Smoothie with banana.

Lunch: Turkey and avocado wrap with tomato and lettuce.

Dinner: Baked chicken breast with roasted cauliflower and asparagus.

Snack: Celery sticks with peanut butter.

Day 8:

Breakfast: Oatmeal with almond milk, chia seeds, and banana.

Lunch: Quinoa and black bean salad with olive oil and lemon juice.

Dinner: Baked salmon with steamed vegetables.

Snack: Greek yogurt with berries.

Day 9:

Breakfast: Avocado toast with a side of scrambled eggs.

Lunch: Lentil soup with a side of steamed vegetables.

Dinner: Baked cod with roasted cauliflower and asparagus.

Snack: Carrot sticks with hummus.

Day 10:

Breakfast: Overnight oats with chia seeds, berries and almond milk.

Lunch: Hummus wrap with lettuce, tomato, and cucumber.

Dinner: Baked turkey with mashed potatoes and green beans.

Snack: Edamame with sea salt.

Day 11:

Breakfast: Egg scramble with bell peppers, onions, and spinach.

Lunch: Tuna salad with cucumber, lettuce, and tomato.

Dinner: Vegetable stir fry with brown rice.

Snack: Apple slices with almond butter.

Day 12:

Breakfast: Granola and fruit-topped Greek yogurt parfait.

Lunch: Grilled turkey sandwich with lettuce and tomato.

Dinner: Baked tilapia with roasted potatoes and Brussels sprouts.

Snack: Celery sticks with peanut butter.

Day 13:

Breakfast: Banana, almond milk, spinach, and protein powder in a smoothie.

Lunch: Chickpea and quinoa salad with olive oil and lemon juice.

Dinner: Green beans and mashed potatoes with roasted turkey breast.

Snack: Greek yogurt with berries.

Day 14:

Breakfast: Egg muffins with spinach, peppers and cheese.

Lunch: Hummus wrap with lettuce, tomato, and cucumber.

Dinner: Baked chicken breast with roasted cauliflower and asparagus.

Snack: Apple slices with almond butter.

Day 15:

Breakfast: Overnight oats with chia seeds, almond milk, and berries.

Lunch: Lentil soup with a side of steamed vegetables.

Dinner: Baked salmon with steamed vegetables.

Snack: Carrot sticks with hummus.

Day 16:

Breakfast: Avocado toast with a side of scrambled eggs.

Lunch: Quinoa and black bean salad with olive oil and lemon juice.

Dinner: Baked cod with roasted cauliflower and asparagus.

Snack: Edamame with sea salt.

Day 17:

Breakfast: Oatmeal with almond milk, chia seeds, and banana.

Lunch: With lettuce and tomato, a turkey and avocado wrap.

Snack: Celery sticks with peanut butter.

Day 18:

Breakfast: Egg scramble with bell peppers, onions, and spinach.

Lunch: Tuna salad with lettuce, tomato, and cucumber.

Dinner: Baked tilapia with roasted potatoes and Brussels sprouts.

Snack: Greek yogurt with berries.

Day 19:

Breakfast: Granola and berries on a Greek yogurt parfait.

Lunch: Grilled turkey sandwich with lettuce and tomato.

Dinner: Baked chicken breast with roasted cauliflower and asparagus.

Snack: Apple slices with almond butter.

Day 20:

Breakfast: Smoothie with banana, almond milk, spinach, and protein powder.

Lunch: Chickpea and quinoa salad with olive oil and lemon juice.

Dinner: Mashed potatoes, green beans, and roasted turkey breast.

Snack: Carrot sticks with hummus.

Day 21:

Breakfast: Egg muffins with spinach, peppers and cheese.

Lunch: Lentil soup with a side of steamed vegetables.

Dinner: Baked salmon with steamed vegetables.

Snack: Edamame with sea salt.

Day 22:

Breakfast: chia seeds, almond milk, and berries in overnight oats.

Lunch: Hummus wrap with lettuce, tomato, and cucumber.

Dinner: Baked cod with roasted cauliflower and asparagus.

Snack: Celery sticks with peanut butter.

Day 23:

Breakfast: Avocado toast with a side of scrambled eggs.

Lunch: Quinoa and black bean salad with olive oil and lemon juice.

Dinner: Baked turkey with mashed potatoes and green beans.

Snack: Greek yogurt with berries.

Day 24:

Breakfast: Oatmeal with almond milk, chia seeds, and banana.

Lunch: Turkey and avocado wrap with lettuce and tomato.

Dinner: Vegetable stir fry with brown rice.

Snack: Apple slices with almond butter.

Day 25:

Breakfast: Egg scramble with bell peppers, onions, and spinach.

Lunch: Tuna salad with lettuce, tomato, and cucumber.

Dinner: Baked tilapia with roasted potatoes and Brussels sprouts.

Snack: Carrot sticks with hummus.

Day 26:

Breakfast: Greek yogurt parfait with granola and berries.

Lunch: Grilled turkey sandwich with lettuce and tomato.

Dinner: Baked chicken breast with roasted cauliflower and asparagus.

Snack: Edamame with sea salt.

Day 27:

Breakfast: Smoothie with banana, almond milk, spinach, and protein powder.

Lunch: Chickpea and quinoa salad with olive oil and lemon juice.

Dinner: Roasted turkey breast with mashed potatoes and green beans.

Snack: Celery sticks with peanut butter.

Day 28:

Breakfast: Egg muffins with spinach, peppers and cheese.

Lunch: Lentil soup with a side of steamed vegetables.

Dinner: Baked salmon with steamed vegetables.

Snack: Greek yogurt with berries.

Day 29:

Breakfast: Overnight oats with chia seeds, almond milk, and berries.

Lunch: Hummus wrap with lettuce, tomato, and cucumber.

Dinner: Baked cod with roasted cauliflower and asparagus.

Snack: Apple slices with almond butter.

Day 30:

Breakfast: Avocado toast with a side of scrambled eggs.

Lunch: Quinoa and black bean salad with olive oil and lemon juice.

Dinner: Baked turkey with mashed potatoes and green beans.

Snack: Carrot sticks with hummus.

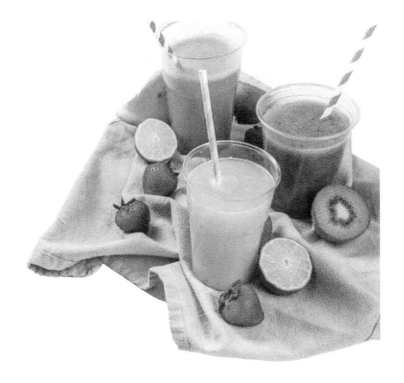

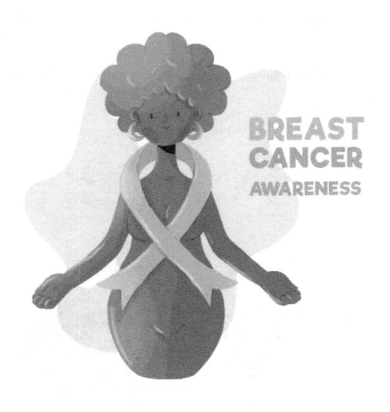

Conclusion

The importance of a breast cancer diet is significant for those who have been newly diagnosed. Eating healthy foods, following a proper nutrition plan, and maintaining a balanced lifestyle can all help to reduce the risk of recurrence and improve overall health outcomes. Here are seven reasons why a breast cancer diet is beneficial:

1. A healthy diet can help reduce the risk of recurrence. Eating fresh and nutrient-rich foods can help to reduce inflammation, improve the body's response to treatments, and reduce the risk of recurrence.

2. Eating nutrient-rich foods can help to boost the immune system. Eating fruits, vegetables, and other sources of antioxidants can help to strengthen the immune system and fight inflammation.

3. Eating healthy foods can reduce the risk of developing other forms of cancer. Eating a diet high in fiber, low in

saturated fat, and with plenty of fruits and vegetables can reduce the risk of developing other forms of cancer.

4. Eating healthy can help to reduce the risk of heart disease. Eating a diet rich in omega-3 fatty acids, fruits, vegetables, and whole grains can help to reduce the risk of developing heart disease.

5. Eating a balanced diet can help to maintain a healthy weight. Eating a diet that is high in fiber, low in saturated fat, and with plenty of fruits and vegetables can help to maintain a healthy weight.

6. Eating healthy foods can provide the body with essential vitamins and minerals. Eating nutrient-rich foods such as fruits, vegetables, and whole grains can help to provide the body with essential vitamins and minerals.

7. Eating healthy can help to reduce stress and improve mental health. Eating a balanced diet and getting enough physical activity can help to reduce stress and improve mental health.

These are just a few of the reasons why a breast cancer diet is essential for those who have been recently diagnosed. Eating the right foods and following a proper nutrition plan can help to reduce the risk of recurrence, boost the immune system, reduce the risk of developing other forms of cancer, and improve overall health.

Moving forward with a healthy lifestyle is key for those who have been newly diagnosed with breast cancer. Eating a balanced diet, exercising regularly, and getting enough rest can all help to reduce the risk of recurrence and improve overall health. Additionally, managing stress and maintaining strong social connections can help to improve mental health and emotional well-being.

When it comes to eating healthy, it is important to consult with a registered dietitian or nutritionist to ensure that you are getting the necessary nutrients your body needs. They can help to create a personalized nutrition plan that is tailored to your individual needs.

Ultimately, by following the tips outlined in this breast cancer diet cookbook and maintaining a healthy lifestyle, those who have been newly diagnosed with breast cancer can reduce the risk of recurrence and improve overall health outcomes. Eating healthy, exercising regularly, and managing stress can all help to make a positive difference in the life of someone who has been newly diagnosed with breast cancer.

Made in the USA
Monee, IL
22 April 2025

16195521R10085